FOR NURSING AND HEALTH PROFESSIONALS

DRUG INDEX NOTE BOOK

FIRST EDITION

Learning and identifying drugs made easy.

AF730419

DR ANNAH SHINGIRAI PARAFFIN

PHD, MNurs, MAgSt, BNurs, BscAg, GCert Nurs, CN.

EMINENCE SKILLS

Email: annah@eminenceskills.com

Website: www.eminenceskills.com

ISBN: 978 - 1 - 7642078-0-5

Cover design and layout – Print Graphics Co

PREFACE

This book helps students to easily identify medications commonly used in the healthcare and veterinary settings. It is designed to simplify documentation and systematic drug research and to aid knowledge retention. The pocket-size, is appropriate for use by students on clinical placements or internships from nursing, pharmacology, paramedicine, veterinary nursing, medical and physiotherapy fraternities.

DEDICATION

This index book is dedicated to my daughter Kathyrn. I believe the simple concepts shared here will help you learn drugs easily. You will not know all drugs in one go. No one does. However, if you choose to study and only learn two to three drugs per day, you will be amazed by what you will know at the end of your placements. The simple act of writing down the name of the drug, its class and indication will help you with knowledge retention.

Let's get started!

-Success Quote-

“You know it may be hard, but you believe you can learn just about anything when you put your mind to it and put your time into it“.

Carol Dweck

MEDICAL TERMS AND ABBREVIATIONS

MEDICAL TERMS AND ABBREVIATIONS

Abbr.	Meaning
AAA	Abdominal aortic aneurysm
ABG	Arterial Blood Gases
ABI	Acquired Brain Injury
ACAT	Aged care assessment team
ACE	Angiotensin converting enzyme
ACS	Acute Coronary Syndrome
AF	Atrial fibrillation
ADL	Activities of daily living
AMI	Acute myocardial infarct
AVR	Aortic valve replacement
APTT	Activated Partial Thromboplastin Time
BGL	Blood Glucose level

BIPAP	Bi- level possible airway pressure
BIBA	Brought in by Ambulance
BP	Blood pressure
BMI	Body Mass Index
CABG	Coronary Artery Bypass Graft
CCF	Congestive/chronic heart failure
CPAP	Continuous positive airway pressure
COPD	Chronic obstructive pulmonary disease
CRP	C-reactive protein
CT	Computed tomography
CKD	Chronic kidney disease
CVD	Cerebrovascular disease
CVAD	Central venous access device
DD	Dangerous drug

DOA	Dead on arrival
DVT	Deep vein thrombosis
ECG	Electrocardiogram
eGFR	Estimated glomerular filtration rate
EF	Ejection Fraction
EST	Exercise Stress Test
ENT	Ear Nose and Throat
EOL	End of life
FBC	Full blood count
GCS	Glasgow Coma scale
GFR	Glomerular filtration rate
GORD	Gastroesophageal reflux disease
GTT	Glucose Tolerance Test
HDL	High density lipoprotein
HEHP	High energy high protein

HITH	Hospital in the home
HPU	Has passed urine
HTN	Hypertension
ICC	Intercostal catheter
ICD	Implantable Cardiac Defibrillator
IDC	Indwelling catheter
IHD	Ischaemic heart disease
INR	International normalized ratio
IVC	Intravenous cannula
IVT	Intravenous therapy
LBBB	Left bundle branch block
LDL	Low density lipoprotein
LF	Liver failure
LFT	Liver Function Test

LLL	Left Lower Lobe
LUL	Left Upper Lobe
MANE	Morning
MAP	Mean Arterial Pressure
MI	Myocardial Infarct
MS	Mitral Stenosis
MRSA	Methicillin Resistant Staphylococcus Aureus
MSU	Mid-Stream Urine
MVA	Motor Vehicle Accident
NG	Nasogastric tube
NSTEMI	Non-ST Elevation Myocardial Infarct
NOCTE	Night
N	Non-steroidal anti-inflammatory drug
PAC	Pressure area care

PCI	Percutaneous Coronary Intervention
PE	Pulmonary Embolus
PICC	Peripherally Inserted Central Catheter
PPE	Personal Protective Equipment
PPM	Permanent Pacemaker
PND	Paroxysmal Nocturnal Dyspnoea
PO	Per oral
PU	Passed urine
PUIT	Passed urine in toilet
PVD	Peripheral Vascular Disease
QID	Four times per Day
SAM	Systolic Anterior Motion
SB	Sinus Bradycardia
SOB	Shortness of Breath
STEMI	ST Elevation MI

TAVI	Trans Aortic Valve Implant
TIA	Transient Ischaemic Attack
TGA	Transposition of the Great Arteries
TOE	Transoesophageal Echo
TOF	Tetralogy of Fallot
TTE	Transthoracic Echo
TV	Tidal Volume
TVD	Triple Vessel Disease
T2DM	Type 2 diabetes Mellitus
UTI	Urinary Tract Infection
VAD	Ventricular Assist Device
VRE	Vancomycin Resistant Enterococci
VSD	Ventricular Septal Defect
VF	Ventricular Fibrillation
VT	Ventricular Tachycardia

MEDICATION AFFIXES

MEDICATION AFFIXES

You can easily identify drug classes by their prefixes and suffixes. The table below lists some commonly used drugs in hospitals or veterinary clinics.

Affixes and Drug class	Mode of action	Common indications	Examples
-lol **Beta Blockers**	Reduce BP by slowing heart rate and reducing myocardial contractility	Hypertension Angina Myocardial infarction Tachyarrhythmia	Metoprolol, Bisoprolol, Atenolol, Nebivolol Carvedilol
-cillin, -mycin -oxacin **Antibiotic/ Anti-infectives**	Inhibit bacterial growth and proliferation	Bacterial infections Pneumonia Wound septicaemia	Flucloxacillin Erythromycin Ciprofloxacin Pipercillin with tazobactam (Piptaz)

-pril **Ace-inhibitors**	Promote dilation of blood vessel, Reduce blood pressure. Prevent conversion of angiotensin 1 to angiotensin 2.	Hypertension Post myocardial infarction. CHF Diabetic nephropathy	Ramipril, Fosinopril, Perindopril Lisinopril, Enalapril, Captopril
-pram -ine **Selective serotonin reuptake inhibitors**	Block or delay the reabsorption of serotonin	Depression Anxiety disorders	Citalopram Escitalopram Fluoxetine Paroxetine Sertraline
-one **Corticosteroid**	Anti-inflammatory	Acute gout Exacerbation of COPD Autoimmune diseases Acute asthma	Dexamethasone Prednisolone Betamethasone Hydrocortisone
-am -pam **Anti-anxiolytic Benzodiazepines**	Reduce anxiety, aid muscle relaxation, sedation	Anxiety Muscle spasm Acute alcohol withdrawal Insomnia	Diazepam, Lorazepam, Oxazepam, Temazepam, Clobazam

-pine **Calcium channel blockers**	Block inward movement of calcium into cells of smooth muscles. Reduce BP	Hypertension Angina	Amlodipine, Nifedipine, Felodipine, Lercanidipine
-prazole **Proton pump inhibitors**	Reduce gastric acid secretion	GORD Reflux Peptic ulcer disease	Pantaprozole, omeprazole, lansoprazole, rabaprazole
-sartan **Angiotensin 2 Receptor blockers**	Inhibit constriction of blood vessels, promote vasodilation and reduce blood pressure	Hypertension	Candesartan, Losartan, Irbesartan, Telmisartan ,Valsartan
-statin **Antilipidemic**	Reduce cholestrol	Hyper-cholesterolaemia Patients at high risk of cardiovascular diseases	Rosuvastattin simvastatin, atorvarstatin

-vir **Antiviral**	Inhibit viral proliferation, inhibit synthesis of viral DNA polymerase and DNA synthesis	Treatment and prevention of herpessimplex infections Shingles Treatment and prevention CMV disease after organ transplant.	Acyclovir Ganciclovir, Valaciclovir
-terol **Bronchodilators**	Dilate bronchi and bronchioles reducing resistance in airway and increasing airflow to the lungs	Asthma COPD	Salmeterol Formoterol
-parin -ran -rin **Anticoagulants**	Inactivation of clotting factors	Prevention of VTE and DVT Acute stemi, non-stemi and unstable angina	Enoxaparin Heparin Dabigatran Warfarin

-actone **Potassium sparing diuretics**	Increase excretion of fluids or water from the kidney. Aid in retention of potassium	CCF CHF	Spironolactone Aldactone
-ase **Thrombolytics**	Break down clots	Acute stemi Pulmonary embolism Acute ischaemic stroke	Alteplase
-zine **Antihistamine**	Reduce the effects of histamines by binding to the H1 receptors	Allergic conditions Rhinitis Itch Sedation Nausea and vomiting	Cyclizine Promethazine Doxylamine
-lax **Laxatives**	Stool softening and promotion of evacuation of faeces	Constipation Faecal impaction Bowel prep before surgery Hepatic encephalopathy	Actilax Dulcolax Microlax Movicol

-caines **Local anaesthetics & Antiarrhythmic agents**	Prevent the transmission of nerve impulses or pain	Iv regional anathesia, nerve block, epidural analgesia Treatment of serious ventricular arrthymias	Lidocaine Lignocaine Xylocaine
-tidine **H2-receptor antagonists**	Reduce production of stomach acid and blocks the action histamine in the gut	GORD Reflux Peptic ulcer disease	Famotidine Ranitidine
-phylline **Bronchodilators**	Enhance dilation of bronchi and bronchioles reduce resistance in the airways and increasing airflow in the lungs	Asthma COPD	Theophylline

(Source: Australian Medicines Handbook, 2025.)

Let's get Learning...

A

Name of drug:

Class:

Mode of action:

Indication:

Name of drug:

Class:

Mode of action:

Indication:

Name of drug:

Class:

Mode of action:

Indication:

Name of drug:

Class:

Mode of action:

Indication:

Name of drug:

Class:

Mode of action:

Indication:

Name of drug:

Class:

Mode of action:

Indication:

A

Name of drug:

Class:

Mode of action:

Indication:

Name of drug:

Class:

Mode of action:

Indication:

Name of drug:

Class:

Mode of action:

Indication:

Name of drug:

Class:

Mode of action:

Indication:

Name of drug:

Class:

Mode of action:

Indication:

Name of drug:

Class:

Mode of action:

Indication:

Name of drug: A

Class:

Mode of action:

Indication:

Name of drug:

Class:

Mode of action:

Indication:

Name of drug:

Class:

Mode of action:

Indication:

Name of drug:

Class:

Mode of action:

Indication:

Name of drug:

Class:

Mode of action:

Indication:

Name of drug:

Class:

Mode of action:

Indication:

Name of drug:

Class: B

Mode of action:

Indication:

Name of drug:

Class:

Mode of action:

Indication:

Name of drug:

Class:

Mode of action:

Indication:

Name of drug:

Class:

Mode of action:

Indication:

Name of drug:

Class:

Mode of action:

Indication:

Name of drug:

Class:

Mode of action:

Indication:

Name of drug:

Class:

Mode of action:

Indication:

Name of drug:

Class:

Mode of action:

Indication:

Name of drug:

Class:

Mode of action:

Indication:

Name of drug:

Class:

Mode of action:

Indication:

Name of drug:

Class:

Mode of action:

Indication:

Name of drug:

Class:

Mode of action:

Indication:

Name of drug:

Class: B

Mode of action:

Indication:

Name of drug:

Class:

Mode of action:

Indication:

Name of drug:

Class:

Mode of action:

Indication:

Name of drug:

Class:

Mode of action:

Indication:

Name of drug:

Class:

Mode of action:

Indication:

Name of drug:

Class:

Mode of action:

Indication:

Name of drug:

Class:

Mode of action:

C

Indication:

Name of drug:

Class:

Mode of action:

Indication:

Name of drug:

Class:

Mode of action:

Indication:

Name of drug:

Class:

Mode of action:

Indication:

Name of drug:

Class:

Mode of action:

Indication:

Name of drug:

Class:

Mode of action:

Indication:

Name of drug:

Class:

Mode of action:

C

Indication:

Name of drug:

Class:

Mode of action:

Indication:

Name of drug:

Class:

Mode of action:

Indication:

Name of drug:

Class:

Mode of action:

Indication:

Name of drug:

Class:

Mode of action:

Indication:

Name of drug:

Class:

Mode of action:

Indication:

Name of drug:

Class:

Mode of action: C

Indication:

Name of drug:

Class:

Mode of action:

Indication:

Name of drug:

Class:

Mode of action:

Indication:

Name of drug:

Class:

Mode of action:

Indication:

Name of drug:

Class:

Mode of action:

Indication:

Name of drug:

Class:

Mode of action:

Indication:

Name of drug:

Class:

Mode of action:

D

Indication:

Name of drug:

Class:

Mode of action:

Indication:

Name of drug:

Class:

Mode of action:

Indication:

Name of drug:

Class:

Mode of action:

Indication:

Name of drug:

Class:

Mode of action:

Indication:

Name of drug:

Class:

Mode of action:

Indication:

Name of drug:

Class:

Mode of action:

D

Indication:

Name of drug:

Class:

Mode of action:

Indication:

Name of drug:

Class:

Mode of action:

Indication:

Name of drug:

Class:

Mode of action:

Indication:

Name of drug:

Class:

Mode of action:

Indication:

Name of drug:

Class:

Mode of action:

Indication:

Name of drug:

Class:

Mode of action:

D

Indication:

Name of drug:

Class:

Mode of action:

Indication:

Name of drug:

Class:

Mode of action:

Indication:

Name of drug:

Class:

Mode of action:

Indication:

Name of drug:

Class:

Mode of action:

Indication:

Name of drug:

Class:

Mode of action:

Indication:

Name of drug:

Class:

Mode of action:

E

Indication:

Name of drug:

Class:

Mode of action:

Indication:

Name of drug:

Class:

Mode of action:

Indication:

Name of drug:

Class:

Mode of action:

Indication:

Name of drug:

Class:

Mode of action:

Indication:

Name of drug:

Class:

Mode of action:

Indication:

Name of drug:

Class:

Mode of action:

E

Indication:

Name of drug:

Class:

Mode of action:

Indication:

Name of drug:

Class:

Mode of action:

Indication:

Name of drug:

Class:

Mode of action:

Indication:

Name of drug:

Class:

Mode of action:

Indication:

Name of drug:

Class:

Mode of action:

Indication:

Name of drug:

Class:

Mode of action:

E

Indication:

Name of drug:

Class:

Mode of action:

Indication:

Name of drug:

Class:

Mode of action:

Indication:

Name of drug:

Class:

Mode of action:

Indication:

Name of drug:

Class:

Mode of action:

Indication:

Name of drug:

Class:

Mode of action:

Indication:

Name of drug:

Class:

Mode of action:

F

Indication:

Name of drug:

Class:

Mode of action:

Indication:

Name of drug:

Class:

Mode of action:

Indication:

Name of drug:

Class:

Mode of action:

Indication:

Name of drug:

Class:

Mode of action:

Indication:

Name of drug:

Class:

Mode of action:

Indication:

Name of drug:

Class:

Mode of action:

F

Indication:

Name of drug:

Class:

Mode of action:

Indication:

Name of drug:

Class:

Mode of action:

Indication:

Name of drug:

Class:

Mode of action:

Indication:

Name of drug:

Class:

Mode of action:

Indication:

Name of drug:

Class:

Mode of action:

Indication:

Name of drug:

Class:

Mode of action:

F

Indication:

Name of drug:

Class:

Mode of action:

Indication:

Name of drug:

Class:

Mode of action:

Indication:

Name of drug:

Class:

Mode of action:

Indication:

Name of drug:

Class:

Mode of action:

Indication:

Name of drug:

Class:

Mode of action:

Indication:

Let's simplify the terms!

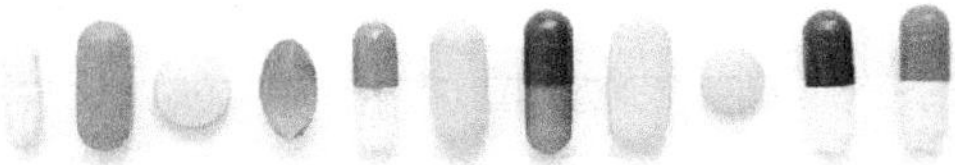

- **Analgesics -** relieve pain. The non-narcotic analgesics are used for treatment of mild pain, and narcotic analgesics or opioids are used for acute and severe pain.
- **Antacids -** relieve indigestion and heartburn by neutralizing stomach acid.
- **Anti-anxiolytics -** suppress anxiety and relax muscles and sometimes used for the sedative effects.
- **Antiarrhythmics -** control irregularities of heartbeat.
- **Antibacterials** - treat bacterial infections.
- **Anticoagulants** - prevent blood from clotting.
- **Thrombolytics** - help dissolve and disperse blood clots and may be prescribed for patients with recent arterial or venous thrombosis.
- **Anticonvulsants** - prevent epileptic seizures.

Name of drug:

Class:

Mode of action:

Indication:

Name of drug:

Class:

Mode of action:

Indication:

Name of drug:

Class:

Mode of action:

Indication:

Name of drug:

Class:

Mode of action:

Indication:

G

Name of drug:

Class:

Mode of action:

Indication:

Name of drug:

Class:

Mode of action:

Indication:

Name of drug:

Class:

Mode of action:

Indication:

Name of drug:

Class:

Mode of action:

Indication:

Name of drug:

Class:

Mode of action:

Indication:

Name of drug:

Class:

Mode of action:

Indication:

G

Name of drug:

Class:

Mode of action:

Indication:

Name of drug:

Class:

Mode of action:

Indication:

Name of drug:

Class:

Mode of action:

Indication:

Name of drug:

Class:

Mode of action:

Indication:

Name of drug:

Class:

Mode of action:

Indication:

Name of drug:

Class:

Mode of action:

Indication:

G

Name of drug:

Class:

Mode of action:

Indication:

Name of drug:

Class:

Mode of action:

Indication:

Name of drug:

Class:

Mode of action:

Indication:

Name of drug:

Class:

Mode of action:

Indication:

Name of drug:

Class:

Mode of action:

Indication:

Name of drug:

Class:

Mode of action:

Indication:

H

Name of drug:

Class:

Mode of action:

Indication:

Name of drug:

Class:

Mode of action:

Indication:

Name of drug:

Class:

Mode of action:

Indication:

Name of drug:

Class:

Mode of action:

Indication:

Name of drug:

Class:

Mode of action:

Indication:

Name of drug:

Class:

Mode of action:

Indication:

H

Name of drug:

Class:

Mode of action:

Indication:

Name of drug:

Class:

Mode of action:

Indication:

Name of drug:

Class:

Mode of action:

Indication:

Name of drug:

Class:

Mode of action:

Indication:

Name of drug:

Class:

Mode of action:

Indication:

Name of drug:

Class:

Mode of action:

Indication:

H

Name of drug:

Class:

Mode of action:

Indication:

Name of drug:

Class:

Mode of action:

Indication:

Name of drug:

Class:

Mode of action:

Indication:

Name of drug:

Class:

Mode of action:

Indication:

Name of drug:

Class:

Mode of action:

Indication:

Name of drug:

Class:

Mode of action:

Indication:

Name of drug:

Class:

Mode of action:

Indication:

Name of drug:

Class:

Mode of action:

Indication:

Name of drug:

Class:

Mode of action:

Indication:

Name of drug:

Class:

Mode of action:

Indication:

Name of drug:

Class:

Mode of action:

Indication:

Name of drug:

Class:

Mode of action:

Indication:

Name of drug:

Class:

Mode of action:

Indication:

Name of drug:

Class:

Mode of action:

Indication:

Name of drug:

Class:

Mode of action:

Indication:

Name of drug:

Class:

Mode of action:

Indication:

Name of drug:

Class:

Mode of action:

Indication:

Name of drug:

Class:

Mode of action:

Indication:

Name of drug:

Class:

Mode of action:

Indication:

Name of drug:

Class:

Mode of action:

Indication:

Name of drug:

Class:

Mode of action:

Indication:

Name of drug:

Class:

Mode of action:

Indication:

Name of drug:

Class:

Mode of action:

Indication:

Name of drug:

Class:

Mode of action:

Indication:

Name of drug: J

Class:

Mode of action:

Indication:

Name of drug:

Class:

Mode of action:

Indication:

Name of drug:

Class:

Mode of action:

Indication:

Name of drug:

Class:

Mode of action:

Indication:

Name of drug:

Class:

Mode of action:

Indication:

Name of drug:

Class:

Mode of action:

Indication:

Name of drug:

Class:

Mode of action:

Indication:

Name of drug:

Class:

Mode of action:

Indication:

Name of drug:

Class:

Mode of action:

Indication:

Name of drug:

Class:

Mode of action:

Indication:

Name of drug:

Class:

Mode of action:

Indication:

Name of drug:

Class:

Mode of action:

Indication:

Name of drug:

Class:

Mode of action:

Indication:

Name of drug:

Class:

Mode of action:

Indication:

Name of drug:

Class:

Mode of action:

Indication:

Name of drug:

Class:

Mode of action:

Indication:

Name of drug:

Class:

Mode of action:

Indication:

Name of drug:

Class:

Mode of action:

Indication:

Name of drug:

Class: K

Mode of action:

Indication:

Name of drug:

Class:

Mode of action:

Indication:

Name of drug:

Class:

Mode of action:

Indication:

Name of drug:

Class:

Mode of action:

Indication:

Name of drug:

Class:

Mode of action:

Indication:

Name of drug:

Class:

Mode of action:

Indication:

Name of drug:

Class:

K

Mode of action:

Indication:

Name of drug:

Class:

Mode of action:

Indication:

Name of drug:

Class:

Mode of action:

Indication:

Name of drug:

Class:

Mode of action:

Indication:

Name of drug:

Class:

Mode of action:

Indication:

Name of drug:

Class:

Mode of action:

Indication:

Name of drug:

Class: K

Mode of action:

Indication:

Name of drug:

Class:

Mode of action:

Indication:

Name of drug:

Class:

Mode of action:

Indication:

Name of drug:

Class:

Mode of action:

Indication:

Name of drug:

Class:

Mode of action:

Indication:

Name of drug:

Class:

Mode of action:

Indication:

Name of drug:

Class:

Mode of action: L

Indication:

Name of drug:

Class:

Mode of action:

Indication:

Name of drug:

Class:

Mode of action:

Indication:

Name of drug:

Class:

Mode of action:

Indication:

Name of drug:

Class:

Mode of action:

Indication:

Name of drug:

Class:

Mode of action:

Indication:

Name of drug:

Class:

Mode of action: L

Indication:

Name of drug:

Class:

Mode of action:

Indication:

Name of drug:

Class:

Mode of action:

Indication:

Name of drug:

Class:

Mode of action:

Indication:

Name of drug:

Class:

Mode of action:

Indication:

Name of drug:

Class:

Mode of action:

Indication:

Name of drug:

Class:

Mode of action:

L

Indication:

Name of drug:

Class:

Mode of action:

Indication:

Name of drug:

Class:

Mode of action:

Indication:

Name of drug:

Class:

Mode of action:

Indication:

Name of drug:

Class:

Mode of action:

Indication:

Name of drug:

Class:

Mode of action:

Indication:

Name of drug:

Class:

Mode of action:

M

Indication:

Name of drug:

Class:

Mode of action:

Indication:

Name of drug:

Class:

Mode of action:

Indication:

Name of drug:

Class:

Mode of action:

Indication:

Name of drug:

Class:

Mode of action:

Indication:

Name of drug:

Class:

Mode of action:

Indication:

Name of drug:

Class:

Mode of action:

M

Indication:

Name of drug:

Class:

Mode of action:

Indication:

Name of drug:

Class:

Mode of action:

Indication:

Name of drug:

Class:

Mode of action:

Indication:

Name of drug:

Class:

Mode of action:

Indication:

Name of drug:

Class:

Mode of action:

Indication:

Name of drug:

Class:

Mode of action:

M

Indication:

Name of drug:

Class:

Mode of action:

Indication:

Let's simplify the terms!

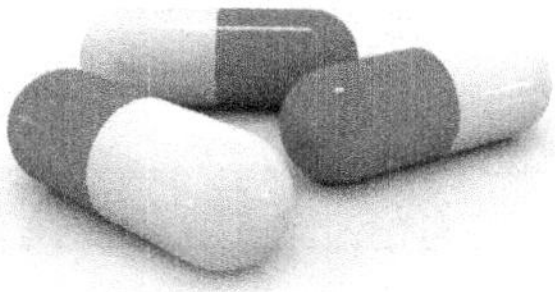

- **Antidepressants -** used for mood-lifting tricyclics, monoamine oxidase inhibitors, and selective serotonin reuptake inhibitors (SSRIs).
- **Antidiarrheals -** relieve diarrhoea. These work in different ways for example by absorbing substances or by slow down bowel muscle contraction.
- **Antiemetics** - treat nausea and vomiting.
- **Antifungals** - treat fungal infections.
- **Antihypertensives** - lower blood pressure.
- **Anti-Inflammatories** - reduce inflammation - the redness, swelling etc.
- **Antineoplastics** - treat cancer.
- **Antipsychotics**- treat symptoms of severe psychiatric disorders.
- **Antipyretics -** reduce fever.

Name of drug:

Class:

Mode of action:

Indication:

Name of drug:

Class:

Mode of action:

N

Indication:

Name of drug:

Class:

Mode of action:

Indication:

Name of drug:

Class:

Mode of action:

Indication:

Name of drug:

Class:

Mode of action:

Indication:

Name of drug:

Class:

Mode of action:

Indication:

Name of drug:

Class:

Mode of action:

Indication:

Name of drug:

Class:

Mode of action:

N

Indication:

Name of drug:

Class:

Mode of action:

Indication:

Name of drug:

Class:

Mode of action:

Indication:

Name of drug:

Class:

Mode of action:

Indication:

Name of drug:

Class:

Mode of action:

Indication:

Name of drug:

Class:

Mode of action:

Indication:

Name of drug:

Class:

Mode of action:

N

Indication:

Name of drug:

Class:

Mode of action:

Indication:

Name of drug:

Class:

Mode of action:

Indication:

Name of drug:

Class:

Mode of action:

Indication:

Name of drug:

Class:

Mode of action:

Indication:

Name of drug:

Class:

Mode of action:

Indication:

Name of drug:

Class:

Mode of action:

O

Indication:

Name of drug:

Class:

Mode of action:

Indication:

Name of drug:

Class:

Mode of action:

Indication:

Name of drug:

Class:

Mode of action:

Indication:

Name of drug:

Class:

Mode of action:

Indication:

Name of drug:

Class:

Mode of action:

Indication:

Name of drug:

Class:

Mode of action:

O

Indication:

Name of drug:

Class:

Mode of action:

Indication:

Name of drug:

Class:

Mode of action:

Indication:

Name of drug:

Class:

Mode of action:

Indication:

Name of drug:

Class:

Mode of action:

Indication:

Name of drug:

Class:

Mode of action:

Indication:

Name of drug:

Class:

Mode of action:

O

Indication:

Name of drug:

Class:

Mode of action:

Indication:

Name of drug:

Class:

Mode of action:

Indication:

Name of drug:

Class:

Mode of action:

Indication:

Name of drug:

Class:

Mode of action:

Indication:

Name of drug:

Class:

Mode of action:

Indication:

Name of drug:

Class:

Mode of action:

Indication:

P

Name of drug:

Class:

Mode of action:

Indication:

Name of drug:

Class:

Mode of action:

Indication:

Name of drug:

Class:

Mode of action:

Indication:

Name of drug:

Class:

Mode of action:

Indication:

Name of drug:

Class:

Mode of action:

Indication:

Name of drug:

Class:

Mode of action:

Indication: P

Name of drug:

Class:

Mode of action:

Indication:

Name of drug:

Class:

Mode of action:

Indication:

Name of drug:

Class:

Mode of action:

Indication:

Name of drug:

Class:

Mode of action:

Indication:

Name of drug:

Class:

Mode of action:

Indication:

Name of drug:

Class:

Mode of action:

Indication:

P

Name of drug:

Class:

Mode of action:

Indication:

Name of drug:

Class:

Mode of action:

Indication:

Name of drug:

Class:

Mode of action:

Indication:

Name of drug:

Class:

Mode of action:

Indication:

Name of drug:

Class:

Mode of action:

Indication:

Name of drug:

Class:

Mode of action:

Indication:

Q

Name of drug:

Class:

Mode of action:

Indication:

Name of drug:

Class:

Mode of action:

Indication:

Name of drug:

Class:

Mode of action:

Indication:

Name of drug:

Class:

Mode of action:

Indication:

Name of drug:

Class:

Mode of action:

Indication:

Name of drug:

Class:

Mode of action:

Indication:

Q

Name of drug:

Class:

Mode of action:

Indication:

Name of drug:

Class:

Mode of action:

Indication:

Name of drug:

Class:

Mode of action:

Indication:

Name of drug:

Class:

Mode of action:

Indication:

Name of drug:

Class:

Mode of action:

Indication:

Name of drug:

Class:

Mode of action:

Indication:

Q

Name of drug:

Class:

Mode of action:

Indication:

Name of drug:

Class:

Mode of action:

Indication:

Name of drug:

Class:

Mode of action:

Indication:

Name of drug:

Class:

Mode of action:

Indication:

Name of drug:

Class:

Mode of action:

Indication:

Name of drug:

Class:

Mode of action:

Indication:

R

Name of drug:

Class:

Mode of action:

Indication:

Name of drug:

Class:

Mode of action:

Indication:

Name of drug:

Class:

Mode of action:

Indication:

Name of drug:

Class:

Mode of action:

Indication:

Name of drug:

Class:

Mode of action:

Indication:

Name of drug:

Class:

Mode of action:

Indication:

Name of drug:

Class:

Mode of action:

Indication:

Name of drug:

Class:

Mode of action:

Indication:

Name of drug:

Class:

Mode of action:

Indication:

Name of drug:

Class:

Mode of action:

Indication:

Name of drug:

Class:

Mode of action:

Indication:

Name of drug:

Class:

Mode of action:

Indication:

R

Name of drug:

Class:

Mode of action:

Indication:

Name of drug:

Class:

Mode of action:

Indication:

Name of drug:

Class:

Mode of action:

Indication:

Name of drug:

Class:

Mode of action:

Indication:

Name of drug:

Class:

Mode of action:

Indication:

Name of drug:

Class:

Mode of action:

Indication:

Name of drug: S

Class:

Mode of action:

Indication:

Name of drug:

Class:

Mode of action:

Indication:

Name of drug:

Class:

Mode of action:

Indication:

Name of drug:

Class:

Mode of action:

Indication:

Name of drug:

Class:

Mode of action:

Indication:

Name of drug:

Class:

Mode of action:

Indication:

Name of drug: S

Class:

Mode of action:

Indication:

Name of drug:

Class:

Mode of action:

Indication:

Name of drug:

Class:

Mode of action:

Indication:

Name of drug:

Class:

Mode of action:

Indication:

Name of drug:

Class:

Mode of action:

Indication:

Name of drug:

Class:

Mode of action:

Indication:

Name of drug:

S

Class:

Mode of action:

Indication:

Name of drug:

Class:

Mode of action:

Indication:

Name of drug:

Class:

Mode of action:

Indication:

Name of drug:

Class:

Mode of action:

Indication:

Let's simplify the terms!

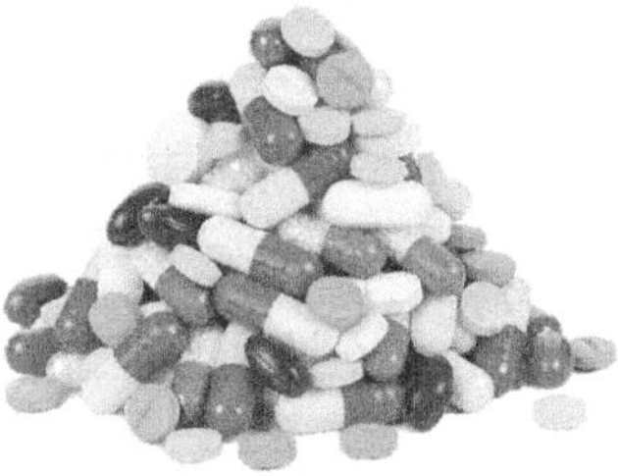

- **Antivirals** - treat viral infections or for prophylaxis against viral infections.
- **Bronchodilators** - open the bronchial tubes and ease breathing
- **Decongestants** - reduce swelling of the mucous membranes by constricting blood vessels, relieving nasal stuffiness.
- **Diuretics** - increase urine production and evacuation of water from the kidneys.
- **Hypoglycemics** – lowers blood glucose.
- **Immunosuppressives** - prevent or reduce the body's normal reaction to invasion by disease or by foreign tissues.
- **Laxatives** - increase the frequency and ease of bowel movements.
- **Vitamins** - chemicals essential in small quantities for good health.

Name of drug:

Class:

Mode of action:

Indication:

Name of drug:

Class:

Mode of action:

Indication:

Name of drug:

Class:

Mode of action:

Indication:

Name of drug:

Class:

Mode of action:

Indication:

Name of drug:

Class:

Mode of action:

Indication:

Name of drug:

Class:

T

Mode of action:

Indication:

Name of drug:

Class:

Mode of action:

Indication:

Name of drug:

Class:

Mode of action:

Indication:

Name of drug:

Class:

Mode of action:

Indication:

Name of drug:

Class:

Mode of action:

Indication:

Name of drug:

Class:

Mode of action:

Indication:

Name of drug:

Class: T

Mode of action:

Indication:

Name of drug:

Class:

Mode of action:

Indication:

Name of drug:

Class:

Mode of action:

Indication:

Name of drug:

Class:

Mode of action:

Indication:

Name of drug:

Class:

Mode of action:

Indication:

Name of drug:

Class:

Mode of action:

Indication:

Name of drug:

Class: T

Mode of action:

Indication:

Name of drug:

Class:

Mode of action:

Indication:

Name of drug:

Class:

Mode of action:

Indication:

Name of drug:

Class:

Mode of action:

Indication:

Name of drug:

Class:

Mode of action:

Indication:

Name of drug:

Class:

Mode of action:

Indication:

Name of drug:

Class:

Mode of action: U

Indication:

Name of drug:

Class:

Mode of action:

Indication:

Name of drug:

Class:

Mode of action:

Indication:

Name of drug:

Class:

Mode of action:

Indication:

Name of drug:

Class:

Mode of action:

Indication:

Name of drug:

Class:

Mode of action:

Indication:

Name of drug:

Class:

Mode of action: U

Indication:

Name of drug:

Class:

Mode of action:

Indication:

Name of drug:

Class:

Mode of action:

Indication:

Name of drug:

Class:

Mode of action:

Indication:

Name of drug:

Class:

Mode of action:

Indication:

Name of drug:

Class:

Mode of action:

Indication:

Name of drug:

Class:

Mode of action:

U

Indication:

Name of drug:

Class:

Mode of action:

Indication:

Name of drug:

Class:

Mode of action:

Indication:

Name of drug:

Class:

Mode of action:

Indication:

Name of drug:

Class:

Mode of action:

Indication:

Name of drug:

Class:

Mode of action:

Indication:

Name of drug:

Class:

Mode of action:

V

Indication:

Name of drug:

Class:

Mode of action:

Indication:

Name of drug:

Class:

Mode of action:

Indication:

Name of drug:

Class:

Mode of action:

Indication:

Name of drug:

Class:

Mode of action:

Indication:

Name of drug:

Class:

Mode of action:

Indication:

Name of drug:

Class:

Mode of action:

V

Indication:

Name of drug:

Class:

Mode of action:

Indication:

Name of drug:

Class:

Mode of action:

Indication:

Name of drug:

Class:

Mode of action:

Indication:

Name of drug:

Class:

Mode of action:

Indication:

Name of drug:

Class:

Mode of action:

Indication:

Name of drug:

Class:

Mode of action:

V

Indication:

Name of drug:

Class:

Mode of action:

Indication:

Name of drug:

Class:

Mode of action:

Indication:

Name of drug:

Class:

Mode of action:

Indication:

Name of drug:

Class:

Mode of action:

Indication:

Name of drug:

Class:

Mode of action:

Indication:

Name of drug:

Class:

Mode of action:

W

Indication:

Name of drug:

Class:

Mode of action:

Indication:

Name of drug:

Class:

Mode of action:

Indication:

Name of drug:

Class:

Mode of action:

Indication:

Name of drug:

Class:

Mode of action:

Indication:

Name of drug:

Class:

Mode of action:

Indication:

Name of drug:

Class:

Mode of action:

Indication:

W

Name of drug:

Class:

Mode of action:

Indication:

Name of drug:

Class:

Mode of action:

Indication:

Name of drug:

Class:

Mode of action:

Indication:

Name of drug:

Class:

Mode of action:

Indication:

Name of drug:

Class:

Mode of action:

Indication:

Name of drug:

Class:

Mode of action:

Indication:

W

Name of drug:

Class:

Mode of action:

Indication:

Name of drug:

Class:

Mode of action:

Indication:

Name of drug:

Class:

Mode of action:

Indication:

Name of drug:

Class:

Mode of action:

Indication:

Name of drug:

Class:

Mode of action:

Indication:

Name of drug:

Class:

Mode of action:

X

Indication:

Name of drug:

Class:

Mode of action:

Indication:

Name of drug:

Class:

Mode of action:

Indication:

Name of drug:

Class:

Mode of action:

Indication:

Name of drug:

Class:

Mode of action:

Indication:

Name of drug:

Class:

Mode of action:

Indication:

Name of drug:

Class:

Mode of action:

X

Indication:

Name of drug:

Class:

Mode of action:

Indication:

Name of drug:

Class:

Mode of action:

Indication:

Name of drug:

Class:

Mode of action:

Indication:

Name of drug:

Class:

Mode of action:

Indication:

Name of drug:

Class:

Mode of action:

Indication:

Name of drug:

Class:

Mode of action:

X

Indication:

Name of drug:

Class:

Mode of action:

Indication:

Name of drug:

Class:

Mode of action:

Indication:

Name of drug:

Class:

Mode of action:

Indication:

Name of drug:

Class:

Mode of action:

Indication:

Name of drug:

Class:

Mode of action:

Indication:

Name of drug:

Class:

Mode of action:

Indication:

Y

Name of drug:

Class:

Mode of action:

Indication:

Name of drug:

Class:

Mode of action:

Indication:

Name of drug:

Class:

Mode of action:

Indication:

Name of drug:

Class:

Mode of action:

Indication:

Name of drug:

Class:

Mode of action:

Indication:

Name of drug:

Class:

Mode of action:

Indication:

Y

Name of drug:

Class:

Mode of action:

Indication:

Name of drug:

Class:

Mode of action:

Indication:

Name of drug:

Class:

Mode of action:

Indication:

Name of drug:

Class:

Mode of action:

Indication:

Name of drug:

Class:

Mode of action:

Indication:

Name of drug:

Class:

Mode of action:

Indication:

Y

Name of drug:

Class:

Mode of action:

Indication:

Name of drug:

Class:

Mode of action:

Indication:

Name of drug:

Class:

Mode of action:

Indication:

Name of drug:

Class:

Mode of action:

Indication:

Name of drug:

Class:

Mode of action:

Indication:

Name of drug:

Class:

Mode of action:

Indication:

Z

Name of drug:

Class:

Mode of action:

Indication:

Name of drug:

Class:

Mode of action:

Indication:

Name of drug:

Class:

Mode of action:

Indication:

Name of drug:

Class:

Mode of action:

Indication:

Name of drug:

Class:

Mode of action:

Indication:

Name of drug:

Class:

Mode of action:

Indication:

Name of drug:

Class:

Mode of action:

Indication:

Name of drug:

Class:

Mode of action:

Indication:

Name of drug:

Class:

Mode of action:

Indication:

Name of drug:

Class:

Mode of action:

Indication:

Name of drug:

Class:

Mode of action:

Indication:

Name of drug:

Class:

Mode of action:

Indication:

Z

Let's wind it up!

-Success Quote-

"Learning never stops, you have to decide and tune your mind to learn".

Dr Annah Paraffin

COMMON DRUG CALCULATIONS FORMULAE TO KNOW

Oral tablets

Dose required = $\frac{Strength\ Required}{Strength\ in\ Stock}$

Liquids, Mixtures and Solutions

Volume Required =

$$\frac{Strength\ Required\ x\ Volume\ of\ Stock\ Solution}{Strength\ in\ Stock}$$

I.V. Rate when asked to infuse over (x) hours

Rate (ml/hr) = $\frac{Volume\ (mls)}{Time\ (hours)x}$

I.V. Rate when asked to infuse over (x) minutes

Rate (ml/hr) = $\frac{Volume\ (mls)\ x\ 60}{Time\ (minutes)}$

I.V infusions using drip rates

Rate (drops/min) = $\frac{Volume\ (mls)\ x\ Drop\ factor}{Time\ (minutes)}$

Concentration of a solution

Concentration (mg/ml) = $\frac{Amount\ of\ drug\ (mg)}{Volume\ (ml)}$

REFERENCES

1. Australian Institute of Health and Welfare. (2019). *Pharmacotherapy in Australia.* Retrieved from https://www.aihw.gov.au/reports/alcohol-other-drug-treatment-services/pharmacotherapy-in-australia
2. Australian Medicines Handbook, 2025. Australian Medicines Handbook Pty Ltd, 2025, Adelaide, Australia
3. McKenna, Lisa & Lim, Anecita Gigi & Mirkov Sanja & adaptation of Karch, Amy Morrison. Pharmacology for nursing and health professional. (2022). McKenna's pharmacology for nursing and health professionals / [Australian and New Zealand adaptation by] Lisa McKenna, Anecita Gigi Lim, Sanja Mirkov; original US edition [by] Amy M. Karch. Macquarie Park, NSW: ©2022: Lippincott Williams & Wilkins
4. Serafini, M., Cargnin, S., Massarotti, A., Tron, G. C., Pirali, T., & Genazzani, A. A. (2021). What's in a Name? Drug Nomenclature and Medicinal Chemistry Trends using INN Publications. *Journal of medicinal chemistry*, *64*(8), 4410–4429. https://doi.org/10.1021/acs.jmedchem.1c00181
5. Tiziani, Adriana. (2022). Havard's nursing guide to drugs / Adriana Tiziani. Chatswood, NSW: Elsevier Australia

Made in the USA
Monee, IL
04 November 2026

67381348R10105